the click guide
to dementia

the click guide to dementia

a **directory** *of* **online resources**
for professionals, carers and individuals
needing care and support

Shirley Ayres
October 2016

About the author

Shirley Ayres is a qualified social worker and marketer who has worked within the care sector for over 35 years. She has extensive experience of helping organisations to understand the power of digital engagement in the social age. Shirley has had a diverse and challenging career in the care sector which has included working with central and local government, charities, the health sector and digital technology start ups.

Shirley now works with organisations excited about the potential of digital technology to transform services and share the learning from success and failure. She is co-founder of the Connected Care Network which promotes collaboration and new partnerships for the digital age.

Shirley is the author of a number of Provocation Papers including *The Long Term Care Revolution* (Innovate UK), *Can online innovations enhance social care?* (Nominet Trust) and *The Future for Personalisation? service users, carers and digital engagement* (Institute for Research and Innovation in Social Services).

She was the co-presenter and producer of The Disruptive Social Care Podcast, a provocative 25 minute weekly video and audio podcast discussing topical issues and events promoting innovations across the care sphere.

blog: shirleyayres.wordpress.com
podcasts: www.disruptivesocialcare.com
twitter: @shirleyayres

Contents

"Technology is a vital part of human existence. They show us that the right tools, in the right hands, can help everyone, regardless of our frailties, to achieve our true potential and advance as a civilisation."

Professor Stephen Hawking accepting his AbilityNet 'Excellence in Accessibility Award' at the Technology4Good Awards, September 2012.

Introduction

Whether you work in the public, private or not-for-profit sectors technology is transforming the way that people connect and services are delivered. Digital technology and social networks provide some of the most powerful tools available today for building a sense of belonging, support and sharing among groups of people who share similar interests and concerns.

Digital technology is driving a revolution in care and the growing use of mobile devices, apps and social networks is becoming significant in enabling people to live more independent lives, irrespective of their health and care needs. Digital technologies provide opportunities to reach out and support people in more exciting and radical ways.

We do need to reassure people that technology will not isolate them further from human contact and community connections. However, it would be wrong not to explore the potential opportunities for enhancing the care and support of people living with dementia and their carers.

The internet is the delivery mechanism for many technology services such as telecare monitoring or online support forums.

At the moment there is no UK wide standard for assessing the effectiveness and quality of health and wellbeing apps unless they are classified as a medical device and regulated by the Medicines and Healthcare Products Regulatory Agency (MHRA). Before downloading an app it is always worth reading Terms and Conditions stating how the data you provide will be stored and checking reviews and star ratings in the Apple and Google App Stores.

Digital technology for social care and wellbeing is a rapidly growing market and to reflect this we are planning to update the Guide in six months.

If your organisation would like to be included in the next edition of the Click Guide to Dementia Resources please provide evidence of your impact via a public link. We will be highlighting those organisations who have shown how they are making a difference to people's lives and the lessons learned from both success and failure.

Social media provides real time feedback and you could show evidence of impact in the following ways: hits on your website, testimonials, downloads of reports, likes and comments on your Facebook page, engagement on Twitter and in discussion forums. As we move towards more open, transparent and accountable organisations we can see publicly if recipients of your services and products have had a positive or negative experience

Please email the details to shirley@clickguide.co.uk with a link to the website and 100 word summary explaining why it should be included.

I hope the Click Guide to Dementia provides many different signposts which enable people to take full advantage of the many online resources available to support people living with dementia, their carers, family and friends.

Overview

Dementia is one of the biggest challenges we face today.
The number of people with Alzheimer's disease, vascular dementia, and other types of dementia is set to double over the next 30 years although some sources suggest that incidence is slowing.

Last year there were 850,000 people with dementia in the UK and according to the Alzheimer's Society, there will be more than one million people living with dementia in the UK by 2025[*].

Research suggests that as many as 30% of residents in extra care housing have mental health problems, most notably dementia. Housing and housing-related services can make the difference between a person with dementia continuing to live independently or moving to a care home. 80 per cent of people living in care homes have a form of dementia or severe memory problems.[†]

In response to these demographics there is a growing range of specialist software and technology to improve the quality of life for the person with dementia, their family, carers and friends through communication, entertainment and stimulation.

Dementia is a broad umbrella term used to describe a range of progressive neurological disorders. There are many different types of dementia and some people may present with a combination of types. Regardless of which type is diagnosed, each person will experience their dementia in their own unique way.

People living with dementia suffer from a variety of conditions ranging from social isolation and depression to behavioural

---

[*] www.nhs.uk/Conditions/dementia-guide/Pages/about-dementia.aspx

[†] www.alzheimers.org.uk/site/scripts/news_article.php?newsID=1498

changes, mood and memory loss. For family and friends there are the additional emotional traumas of being with a person who may not recognise them or remember their shared life. People with dementia may experience spatial and visual challenges as well as the more commonly understood memory issues. Changes in the brain can impact on day to day functions and potentially confuse people living with dementia. Identifying how the home and environment can be modified to ameliorate any challenges will make a difference to the person living with dementia.*

Dementia describes a group of symptoms, such as memory loss, problems with communication skills, reasoning, but also problems with daily tasks, such as cooking and washing. Types of Dementia are for example Alzheimer's disease, Vascular Dementia, Lewy Body Dementia and Frontotemporal Dementia, while Alzheimer's disease is the most common form of Dementia in the UK.

Changes are often small to start with, but for someone with dementia they have become severe enough to affect daily life. How others respond to the person, and how supportive or enabling the person's surroundings are, also greatly affect how well someone can live with dementia.

The health and care sectors are in the early stages of understanding the power and potential of digital technology and social networks to develop new models of support for people living with dementia who may also have other long term conditions and their carers

There are an increasing range of devices and technologies that can make life easier for people with dementia, their carers, families and friends. Technologies and 'apps' (applications or programs for smartphones and tablets) that have been developed for the general

---

* dementia.stir.ac.uk

public are increasingly being used by people with dementia as well. Over time it is possible that these mainstream technologies will replace many of the products that were developed specifically for people with dementia or disability.

Technology can be used in a variety of ways including connected sensors to re-assure or alert family and professional care staff, networks between family and professionals to share information and tasks required to support the person needing care, online forums to support carers, e-marketplaces to help people find information and care services online including purchasing care and devices which make it easier for older people to Skype and use social networks.

There is no doubt that the digital revolution has transformed our daily lives. The emergence and general acceptance of online and digital technologies in our workplaces and homes is a development that has brought positive benefits to millions of people. Using assistive technology has lots of potential benefits but it also has its difficulties. Assistive technology can never replace human contact and interaction. Assistive technology will not eliminate risk. It can only assist people in improving their safety and wellbeing it cannot provide perfect solutions.

It is worth remembering that one size does not fit all and too often we expect that the person will adapt to the technology, not the other way round. Expecting the person with dementia to adapt, without listening to their views, can affect both their willingness and motivation to use the technology. Before rushing for technology solutions it is wise to start by exploring the specific needs, circumstances and aspirations of the individual.

Surprisingly for a person who is a keen advocate of digital technology my first suggestion is to be aware of the value of low tech solutions. Ensuring people live in a safe environment is critical to wellbeing and the simple Magiplug* at a cost of less than £10 prevents baths overflowing using a pressure activated system and picks up if the water temperature is too high.

I hope that the Click Guide to Dementia Resources which brings together innovative resources to support people living with dementia, their families and carers and provides signposts will enable people to make more informed choices about living well with dementia.

Disclaimer

We have made every reasonable effort to ensure that the information contained within the *guide* is accurate. However, the information has been compiled from a number of sources including the websites of the organisations in the *guide*, central and local government bodies, cross referencing and independent research and there may be errors or omissions. Any service, website, helpline, organisation etc. which is mentioned is not an endorsement of that service. Every effort has been made to ensure the accuracy of information given but we cannot accept any liability or responsibility for any errors or omissions. If you are aware of any errors, changes in website addresses etc. please contact us.

---

* www.magiplug.com

Advice, Information and Support

Alzheimer's Society

Alzheimer's Society provide a wide range of services including information and practical and emotional support to help people live well with dementia. They campaign to improve public understanding of dementia and launched the Dementia Friends initiative in November 2012.

There is a Helpline 0300 222 11 22, a live online advice service for dementia information and support and Talking Point an online community for anyone affected by dementia.

The dementia-friendly technology charter has been produced as part of the Dementia Friendly Communities strand of the Prime Minister's challenge on dementia. The charter gives people with dementia and their carers information on how to access technology. It also provides guidance to health, housing and social care professionals on how to make technology work for people based on their individual needs [www.alzheimers.org.uk/technologycharter].

Dementia Connect is the Alzheimer's Society's new and improved dementia services directory for anyone affected by dementia in England, Wales and Northern Ireland. With over 4,000 listings of local information, support and services, it provides an easy-to-use online directory.

website: www.alzheimers.org.uk
facebook: www.alzheimers.org.uk/facebook
twitter: @alzheimerssoc

Alzheimer Society of Ireland

Alzheimer Society of Ireland works across the country in local communities providing dementia specific services and supports and advocating for the rights and needs of all people living with dementia and their carers. The society operates the Alzheimer National Helpline offering information and support to anyone affected by dementia at 1800 341 341 which is open Monday to Friday 10am to 5pm and Saturday 10 am to 4 pm.

website: www.alzheimer.ie
facebook: www.facebook.com/TheAlzheimerSocietyofIreland
twitter: @alzheimersocirl

Alzheimer Scotland

Alzheimer Scotland provides a wide range of specialist services for people with dementia and their carers. They offer personalised support services, community activities, information and advice and a 24 hour Dementia Freephone Helpline 0808 808 3000.

website: www.alzscot.org
facebook: www.facebook.com/AlzheimerScotland
twitter: @alzscot

Alzheimer Europe

Alzheimer Europe is a non-governmental organisation aimed at raising awareness of all forms of dementia by creating a common European platform through co-ordination and co-operation between Alzheimer organisations throughout Europe. Alzheimer Europe is also a source of information on all aspects of dementia.

website: www.alzheimer-europe.org
facebook: www.facebook.com/alzheimer.europe
twitter: @AlzheimerEurope

Alzheimer's Disease International

ADI is the global voice on dementia and the umbrella organisation of Alzheimer associations around the world.

website: alz.co.uk
facebook: www.facebook.com/alzheimersdiseaseinternational
twitter: @AlzDisInt

Dementia Pathfinders

Dementia Pathfinders is a social enterprise delivering education and learning for people working in the dementia care field and providing therapeutic care and support for people with dementia and their families. They seek to build partnerships with individuals and groups working to understand and meet the needs of people with dementia. Projects include hosting the Dementia Roadmap (from 1 April 2015 until 31 March 2018), an online platform providing up-to-date information about dementia diagnosis, treatment and services, to help GPs, nurses and other health and social care professionals deliver the best possible care for people with dementia and their families throughout the dementia 'journey'.

website: dementiapathfinders.org
facebook: www.facebook.com/dementiapathfinders
twitter: @DPCIC

Department of Health

The Department of Health have published an interactive 'dementia atlas' which shows that standards of care vary widely in different areas and critics say has revealed a postcode lottery in care for the chronic and degenerative brain disease.

website: shapeatlas.net/dementia/#6/52.945/-2.147/l-p65
twitter: @DHgovuk

Dementia Alliance International

Dementia Alliance International is a non-profit group of people with dementia from all around the world that seek to represent, support, and educate others living with the disease, and an organization that will provide a unified voice of strength, advocacy and support in the fight for individual autonomy and improved quality of life. Free membership for people with dementia

website: www.dementiaallianceinternational.org
twitter: @DementiaAllianc

Dementia UK

Dementia UK is a charity providing families and people with specialist dementia support and guidance. The unique Admiral Nurses are expert nurses specialising in dementia care who work closely with families, providing support to help them cope with the fear, uncertainty and difficult everyday reality of dementia.

Dementia UK runs a national helpline and email service, called Admiral Nursing Direct, for family and professional carers, people with dementia and those worried about their memory. It is the only nurse-led dementia helpline in the country. The Helpline 0800 888 6678is available from 9:15am to 4.45pm Monday to Friday and also from 6pm to 9pm on Wednesdays and Thursdays.

website: www.dementiauk.org
facebook: www.facebook.com/DementiaUK1
twitter: @DementiaUK

Dementia Society

Dementia Society was founded in 2016 to provide open source materials to improve education in the dementias. The blog offers a focus for discussion of cutting edge policy themes in England and internationally. The "Dementia Rights" project aims to embed through word of mouth and social action a rights based consciousness towards rights.

website: dementiasoc.org.uk
twitter: @dr_shibley

Joseph Rowntree Foundation

Joseph Rowntree Foundation is an independent organisation working to inspire social change through research, policy and practice. The Foundation have explored how dementia will impact the UK and looked at building dementia friendly communities and making cities and organisations dementia friendly.

website: www.jrf.org.uk/people/dementia
facebook: www.facebook.com/JosephRowntreeFoundation
twitter: @jrf_uk

LSE Personal Social Services Research Unit

LSE Personal Social Services Research Unit (PSSRU) have published a dementia toolkit to help patients, carers and healthcare workers. TheDementia Evidence Toolkit is the first of its kind in the world and brings together over 3,000 empirical journal articles and 700 systematic reviews, each of them coded according to type of dementia, care setting, outcome measured, type of intervention and country of study or authors.

website: toolkit.modem-dementia.org.uk
twitter: @MODEMproject

NHS Choices

NHS Choices provides information and advice for people with dementia and their friends and families, including dementia symptoms, diagnosis, treatment, and how to live well. This site offers information for people with dementia and their families and friends. It aims to raise awareness of dementia, as well as help people create networks and better understand the impact of the condition.

Links to information on dementia and sources of local and national support: www.nhs.uk/Conditions/dementia-guide/Pages/dementia-choices.aspx

Staying independent with dementia: www.nhs.uk/conditions/dementia-guide/pages/staying-independent-with-dementia.aspx

Care equipment, aids and adaptations: www.nhs.uk/conditions/social-care-and-support-guide/Pages/equipment-aids-adaptations.aspx

facebook: www.facebook.com/NHSChoices
twitter: @NHSChoices

National Institute for Health and Care Excellence (NICE)

The National Institute for Health and Care Excellence (NICE) provides national guidance and advice to improve health and social care. They provide guidance on a number of dementia topics.

website: www.nice.org.uk

Supporting people with dementia and their carers in health and social care: www.nice.org.uk/Guidance/cg42

facebook: www.facebook.com/NationalInstituteforHealthandCareExcellence
twitter: @NICEcomms

Social Care Institute for Excellence (SCIE)

Social Care Institute for Excellence (SCIE) Dementia Gateway offers a range of helpful resources including information, films, e-Learning resources on dementia, the Mental Capacity Act, restraint and the mental health of older people. The dementia environment at home video shows how simple changes to create a more dementia friendly environment can have a positive impact on a person living with dementia's emotional well being and independence.

website: www.scie.org.uk/dementia
facebook: www.facebook.com/socialcareinstitutepage
twitter: @SCIE_socialcare

YoungDementia UK

YoungDementia UK provides information & support to the more than 40,000 people in the UK with young onset dementia. They are able to offer face-to-face support in the Oxfordshire area.

website: www.youngdementiauk.org
facebook: www.facebook.com/YoungDementiaUK
twitter: @YoungDementiaUK

Blogs and Sharing Experiences

One of the most valuable aspects of social media is the easy access to a wide range of voices sharing experiences of living with dementia and caring for a person with dementia. The dementia community is diverse and flourishing. The following are good examples of individuals using social media to inform, educate and raise awareness.

Professor June Andrews

Professor June Andrews is a Dementia professor and author of Dementia the One Stop Guide which provides practical advice for families, professionals, and people living with dementia and Alzheimer's Disease

blog: juneandrews.net/dementia-the-one-stop-guide
twitter: @ProfJuneAndrews

Beth Britton

Beth Britton is a campaigner, consultant, writer and blogger on ageing, health, social care and dementia.

blog: www.bethbritton.com
twitter: @bethyb1886

Zoe Harris

Zoe Harris is an innovator, social entrepreneur and ex-carer trying to make a difference. She is the founder of @Care_Charts_UK and @Mycarematters

twitter: @ZoeHarrisCCUK

Ming Ho

Ming Ho is a TV and stage writer and dementia campaigner and one of the first to write about dementia and sexual intimacy. Her new play 'The Things We Never Said' which draws on her experience of caring for her mother is coming to BBC R4 in 2017

blog: dementiajustaintsexy.blogspot.co.uk
twitter: @Minghowriter and @neversaidplay

Phillipa Kelly

Phillipa Kelly is a writer and campaigner whose posts about dementia are always poignant and moving.

blog: pippakelly.co.uk
twitter: @piponthecommons

Lucy Marsters

Lucy Marsters is a dementia nurse lead at an NHS Trust.

blog: dementianursedays.blogspot.co.uk
twitter: @lucyjmarsters

Dr Shibley Ramen

Dr Shibley Ramen is passionate about ensuring the public are aware and knowledgeable about current trends in dementia research and how they impact on policy development. Shibley is the author of:

Living well with dementia: the importance of the person and the environment (on amazon.co.uk: http://amzn.to/2dGoAmv)

Living better with dementia: good practice and innovation for the future (on amazon.co.uk: http://amzn.to/2eoai3A)

Enhancing health and wellbeing in dementia: implementing person-centred integrated care (to be published in February 2017)

blog: dementia-wellbeing.org
twitter: @dr_shibley

Sarah Reed

Sarah Reed founded Many Happy Returns as the result of ten years caring for her mother, who lived with Alzheimer's disease and vascular dementia. She developed and published the unique 1940s and 1950s 'Chatterbox' cards to make encounters across the generations more fun and rewarding for everyone involved, through rich, enjoyable conversation. She is the creator of the REAL Communication model.

blog: www.manyhappyreturns.org/our-soaps.html
twitter: @SarahReed_MHR

Chris Roberts

Chris Roberts is living with mixed dementia. Along with his wife @jaynegoodrick and family Chris shared his thoughts and experiences in a powerful BBC Panorama documentary. Pippa Kelly wrote a moving tribute to Chris Roberts here: pippakelly.co.uk/2016/06/chris-roberts-story

video (only in the UK, until 2 December 2016): www.bbc.co.uk/iplayer/episode/b07dxmyh/panorama-living-with-dementia-chriss-story
twitter: @mason423

Kate Swaffer

Kate Swaffer was just 49 years old when she was diagnosed with a form of younger onset dementia. She is the author of *What the Hell Happened to My Brain? Living Beyond Dementia* [available from bookdepository here: http://bit.ly/2dQZ796] which offers an all-too-rare first-hand insight into that experience, sounding a clarion call for change in how we ensure a better quality of life for people with dementia.

twitter: @KateSwaffer

Tommy Whitelaw

Tommy Whitelaw is the project engagement lead for @dementiacarer @ALLIANCEScot. After caring for his mum Joan who had dementia he resolved to use his experiences to improve support for carers.

blog: tommy-on-tour-2011.blogspot.co.uk
twitter: @tommyNtour

Tweetchats

A Twitter tweetchat is a pre-arranged chat that happens on Twitter through the use of Twitter updates (called tweets) and include a predefined hashtag to link those tweets together in a virtual conversation. Formal Twitter tweet chats are arranged in advance and occur at a specific time. Tweetchats can be an easy way to have a discussion and find people across the world who share similar interests and passions.

@AlzChat

@AlzChat host the #AlzChat where Alzheimer's & dementia carers share thoughts, resources and concerns. There is a new topic each week. Founded in 2011 by @irememberbetter with co-host: @creativitycare. The chats take place on Mondays at 8pm GMT.

@DiverseAlz

@DiverseAlz aim to raise dementia awareness in a diverse world where inclusion counts. They host the #Diversealz chat on Thursdays at 8pm GMT.

@Dembkclub

@Dembkclub hosts a tweetchat to discuss books (#Dembk) and blogs (#Demblogs) about dementia on the last Sunday of each month at 8pmGMT.

#AlzAuthors

#AlzAuthors are authors collaborating to provide resources for those living with dementia and their caregivers

blog: alzauthors.wordpress.com

Carer Support Networks

Carers Trust

Carers Trust believe in a world where the role and contribution of unpaid carers is recognised and they have access to the quality support and services they need to live their own lives. They offer online forums for both adult carers and young carers under 18. They also provide a facility to search online for grants and other financial assistance. Carer Smart is a new club from Carers Trust where you can get discounts and cash back. It is open to carers, people with care needs and staff and volunteers across the Carers Trust network.

website: www.carers.org
facebook: www.facebook.com/carerstrust
twitter: @CarersTweets

Carers UK

Carers UK provide an expert telephone advice and support service on 0808 808 7777 (Monday to Friday, 10am to 4pm) and online information and support. This includes benefits and tax credits, carers employment rights, carers' assessment and the services available for carers. The online forum provides a place for carers to share day and night.

website: www.carersuk.org

Digital Resource for Carers

The Digital Resource for Carers brings together a number of digital products and online resources, to help organisations provide comprehensive information and support for carers.

website: www.carersuk.org/for-professionals/carersuk-products/
digital-resource-for-carers

facebook: www.facebook.com/carersuk
twitter: @CarersUK

Chill4usCarers

Chill4usCarers is an independent Forum run by volunteer family Carers and ex carers. Social media is used very actively to raise awareness and support for carers. The Carers' forum provides information, news and views and the online chat room is open 24 hours a day. Chill4usCarers organises Computers4carers which provides free computers for carers.

website: chill4uscarers.co.uk
facebook: www.facebook.com/Chill4usCarers
twitter: @Chill4usCarers

Dementia Carer

Dementia Carer provide resources for carers of people with dementia with tips and hints from carers for carers. The site allows professionals to access a list of the major organisations in their area providing services for carers and people with dementia.

website: www.dementiacarer.net
twitter: @CarerDementia

Dementia Challengers

Dementia Challengers was established by carers for carers to help people access information and advice about dementia. Their website guides carers to online resources including a section on finding the right technology. The Draw Something app a popular social drawing and guessing game.

website: www.dementiachallengers.com
twitter: @dragonmisery

DMAT

The DMAT supports carers to assess, find solutions & create a care plan to enhance mealtime abilities and independence. The aim of the care plan is to create a supportive 'dementia friendly' mealtime environment to enhance the mealtime abilities of someone living with dementia. Using The DMAT can help maintain independence at mealtimes, increase nutritional intake and improve quality of life. Fees are £5/month or £50/year (a one month free trial is offered).

website: thedmat.com
twitter: @TheDMAT

Healthy Living Club

The Healthy Living Club based in Lambeth London, is an inspiring self-directed community group promoting the wellbeing of its members who are people with a dementia, their carers and friends. The group meets weekly to engage in activities chosen to alleviate the symptoms of dementia and/or to help arrest or reverse cognitive decline. All members, including members who would be defined as volunteers at other settings, take part in all activities and enjoy them as much as everybody else. The Healthy Living Club is a joyous example of community support for people living with dementia.

blog: hlclc.wordpress.com
website: healthylivingclub.org.uk
facebook: www.facebook.com/HealthyLivingClubAtLinghamCourt
twitter: @HLCLC

Living Well with Dementia

Living Well with Dementia is an online resource for people affected by dementia living in Warwickshire. The Living Well with Dementia Portal brings together in one place essential advice and resources for people with dementia, their carers, and staff from health and social care. The Coventry and Warwickshire Living Well with Dementia Partnership is dedicated to raising awareness and reducing stigma around dementia.

website: www.livingwellwithdementia.org
twitter: @DementiaCandW

Local authority social care websites will provide information about support for carers in their locality although the quality of information offered can be very variable.

Personal Support Networks

One of the simplest needs for people is the ability to stay in touch with family and friends who may be widely dispersed. There are a range of online tools available to enable connections to be maintained and to address the practical tasks of co-ordinating the care needs of an individual living with dementia.

Technology is being used by personal support networks and Circles of Support to provide safe, moderated online environments which connect family, friends and professionals providing formal and informal care.

There are a number of support networks available and features may include e-mail, a calendar/diary to share tasks and goals, photo sharing, a social network and space to share stories through multi media and text facilities. The software can be available on a web-browser, mobile app and tablet pc. The number of people who can be connected in one network varies. Some networks are free to use and others require a paid subscription. To gain the support of health and care professionals developers need to ensure that there is clear information about how the data that is collected will be secured and used.

Some networks are intended primarily for family and friends and others are aimed at employers, councils, care providers and housing associations.

Mindings

Mindings is a service that enables people to share text messages, personal captioned photos, calendar reminders, and much more, with technology-shy loved ones, on a digital photo frame.

Designed as a light-touch telecare service, Mindings has been described as 'Facebook for the technology-shy', enabling effortless, regular, personal, and meaningful connection.

A single on-screen button sends confirmation and peace-of-mind to the sender that the content has been received.

Mindings is a subscription service that runs on iPad.

website: www.mindings.com
facebook: www.facebook.com/Mindings
twitter: @MindingsStu

Jointly

Developed by Carers UK, the Jointly app is an innovative and cost effective way to support carers by helping them better manage and co-ordinate care. Jointly combines group messaging with other useful features including to-do and medication lists, calendar and more. You can purchase a Jointly circle with an one-off payment of £2.99Available on iPhone, iPad and Android.

website: www.jointlyapp.com

My Care Matters

My Care Matters is a free, secure place online to share information that healthcare professionals need to know about you to provide person centred care. Currently in Beta Version

website: mycarematters.org
twitter: @Mycarematters

Rally Round

Rally Round enables family members, friends and carers to create and organise support for someone they care about. Rally Round was designed to help frail older people and/or their family carers, but it can be used to help anyone who is vulnerable and needs more practical support. Rally Round is free to use and support networks can be started provided the person being helped, or the person starting the network, lives in an area where Rally Round has been made available. Rally Round can be used on any computer, tablet or mobile phone

website: www.rallyroundme.com
twitter: @rallyround1

Cura

Cura is a free online service which makes it easy for friends and family to come together and help a loved one stay safe and well at home. Cura is supported by Cura Homecare Services and can be used on any computer or mobile phone.

website: www.curahq.com

Learning about Dementia

FutureLearn

Whilst there are numerous online courses available these have been recommended because FutureLearn is owned by the Open University who have a worldwide reputation for providing quality online learning and ALISON are one of the top publishers of online learning with over 8 million students.

FutureLearn offer a range of free online courses to help people understand and care for people with dementia. These certificated courses are designed for healthcare professionals or family and friends who care for people with dementia. Developed by leading medical schools and universities, these courses will help you understand the symptoms and challenges associated with dementia, memory loss and Alzheimer's disease, and explore the latest information, research and best practice advice for carers.

website: www.futurelearn.com/courses/collections/dementia
twitter: @FutureLearn

ALISON

ALISON online learning platform provides a free certificated online course Caregiving Skills – Dementia Care designed to ensure people have the skills and knowledge necessary to provide effective care to clients who have been diagnosed with dementia. There are three modules: Understanding the Signs of Dementia, Working with Clients with Different Types of Dementia and Caregiving Skills – Dementia Care.

website: alison.com/courses/caregiving-skills-dementia-care
facebook: www.facebook.com/AdvanceLearning
twitter: @ALISONcourses

SCIE Dementia e-learning course

SCIE Dementia e-learning course is free to use and is aimed at anyone who comes into contact with someone with dementia. It provides a general introduction to the disease and the experience of living with it. This course is designed to be accessible to a wide audience and includes a considerable amount of video footage shot by both the Alzheimer's Society and SCIE where people with dementia and their carers share their views and feelings on camera.

Dementia currently affects around one in six of adults over the age of 80s. With the sad reality that a cure any time soon is unlikely, experts believe that instead of changing the patients themselves, it is time to change the people around them.

website: www.scie.org.uk/dementia/e-learning/index.asp

Virtual Dementia Tour

The Virtual Dementia Tour was designed to not just show people what it is like to have dementia, but also to sense it. An interesting report of experiencing the Dementia simulator.

website: www.ibtimes.co.uk/dementia-simulator-my-experience-virtual-dementia-tour-1538636

Age simulation suit to enhance Dementia Training

The Age Simulation Set combines a system of wearable devices to provide the user with instantaneous simulation of the effects of ageing, and the difficulty associated in mobility with performing every day tasks such as walking, sitting, cooking or answering the phone. Specially devised goggles simulate degraded vision due to cataracts and earplugs reduce hearing ability. Elbow and knee restrictors simulate reduced joint mobility and arm and leg weights simulate weakened muscle power. Wearing the gloves and finger restrictors reduces sense of touch for fingers and the ability to grasp objects making trainee clumsy, while a back brace allows the trainee to experience the stooped posture specific to ageing.

website: www.adam-rouilly.co.uk/news.aspx?id=40

12 Minutes in Alzheimer's Dementia simulation

This video aims   to create awareness and understanding about the impact of living with Alzheimers

website: https://www.youtube.com/watch?v=8eKJwB9ZK5A&utm_content=bufferb07d8&utm_medium=social&utm_source=twitter.com&utm_campaign=buffer

WhoseShoes?

WhoseShoes? is a practical tool helping local authorities, universities, care providers and others move on from the big picture or 'vision' to providing person-centred services for individuals needing care and support. In the form of a thought-provoking board game, Whose Shoes? offers an imaginative, interactive approach. It helps people work together to explore the issues and jointly find a way forward. There are over 200 scenarios which allow real concerns to be raised and discussed. There is also an electronic version of WhoseShoes? Making It Real.

website: www.nutshellcomms.co.uk
facebook: www.facebook.com/whoseshoes.GillPhillips
twitter: @WhoseShoes

Housing and the Home Environment

We all need a better understanding of how to design appropriate buildings and new forms of supported housing which enable people to live well with dementia. Life can change in many ways when someone s diagnosed with dementia. Comfortable and familiar homes can be transformed into a frightening space filled with obstacles. It is important that the design of the living environment responds not only to the needs of the person with dementia but also the carer and wider family. Environmental approaches to reducing both cognitive and behavioural problems associated with dementia are considered critical factors to improving the quality of life for people living with dementia..

HousingLin

The Housing Learning and Improvement Network are at the forefront of connecting people, exchanging ideas and sharing resources to help shape and influence the way we think about and deliver housing with care for an ageing population. In Focus: Innovations in Housing and Dementia provides a range of resources that will help people with dementia to live independently for as long as possible.

website: www.housinglin.org.uk
twitter: @HousingLIN

National Housing Federation

National Housing Federation have published a guide to Dementia Finding housing solutions which highlights examples of good practice from housing associations and home improvement agencies, providing a range of flexible support, specialist housing and home adaptations, which allow people to live well with their condition. The guide recommends that commissioners and their local partners work together with housing organisations to enable people with dementia to retain their independence for as long as possible [www.housinglin.org.uk/_library/Resources/Housing/OtherOrganisation/Dementia_-_Finding_housing_solutions.pdf].

website: www.housing.org.uk
facebook: www.facebook.com/nationalhousingfederation
twitter: @natfednews

Internationally there are an increasing range of housing solutions for people living with dementia.

Hogewey

Hogewey is a gated community in the Netherlands, designed specifically for people with dementia. About 150 people with Alzheimer's or similar live in 23 themed homes where the emphasis is on having as much fun as possible. Hogewey encourages residents to keep up the day-to-day tasks they have always done: gardening, shopping, peeling potatoes, shelling the peas, doing the washing, folding the laundry, going to the hairdresser, popping to the cafe.

Roughly 250 paid healthcare professionals (as well as an unknown number of additional volunteers) assist the residents with most aspects of their lives, but they aren't in traditional lab coats or scrubs, but in regular street clothes. This is all part of the vision of the village to craft a reality around their residents' hopes and desires, rather than constraining them to things they can no longer do with a faltering memory.

website: hogeweyk.dementiavillage.com (use google translate for English version!)

City For Life

Odense Municipality in Denmark has announced plans to build a city district entirely aimed at people with dementia. City For Life will house between 200 and 300 people and provide residents with everything they might need to live out the rest of their lives in a fulfilling way. Odense Municipality are in negotiations to purchase land for City for Life. However, the exact plans for the design of the city and what specific services will be provided are still being discussed. The municipality expects the first residents to move into City for Life at the end of 2018. They are not trying to build a replica of Hogewey but want to create their own version of a township specifically designed for people with dementia.

website: doctordementia.com/2015/06/15/dementia-village-coming-to-denmark

Dementia Enabling Environment Project (DEEP)

Dementia Enabling Environment Project (DEEP) Virtual Information Centre provides practical tips, guides and resources to help make the places where we live more dementia enabling. This will encourage a person with dementia to lead as full and independent life as possible. These can be simple modifications that anybody can make to their home, to landscaping or architectural design changes. Use this site to explore different home settings and learn more about key design principles in each area of the house and to download useful information and resources.

website: www.enablingenvironments.com.au
twitter: @dementiaunited

Dementia Village Advisors

Dementia Village Advisors creates custom living environments for elderly people with dementia which includes Hogewey. They design manageable and pleasant residential areas where it is comfortable for everyone to live and where residents feel safe at home.

website: www.dementiavillage.com
facebook: www.facebook.com/dementiavillage
twitter: @Dementiavillage

YoungDementia UK Homes

YoungDementia UK Homes are planning the first supported living facility in Oxfordshire offering private flats for up to 12 residents.

website: www.youngdementiaukhomes.org
facebook: www.facebook.com
twitter: @YoungDementiaUK

Dementia Services Development Centre

Dementia Services Development Centre has created a 'virtual dementia friendly care home'. This allows a wide range of users to understand and explore design and technology for people with dementia. The Centre currently houses a design and technology suite, which people can visit to gather ideas and advice in terms of design and various aspects of technology for people with dementia. The virtual suite ensures that learning is accessible by all, regardless of where they live or work. The Dementia Centre offer a number of free eBooks available from the online shop.

In Scotland the Centre has published *Improving the design of housing for people with dementia* to raise awareness, explain why particular design features are needed, and to give basic guidance on the most important principles of design [http://bit.ly/2cXW3eK].

Virtual Care Home

The Virtual Care Home is an online resource that demonstrates dementia-friendly design in care home settings or people's own homes. The layouts of seven individual rooms are modelled with information revealed interactively on how the features can make a difference for people living with dementia.

website: dementia.stir.ac.uk/virtualhome
twitter: @dementiacentre

Dementia-Friendly Home

From Australia the Dementia-Friendly Home is designed to help carers adapt or design a home for a person living with dementia. Carers are placed in a virtual home that they can explore at their own pace, learning how to make it more suitable for people with dementia. Each object within the home is interactive, allowing carers to immediately see and hear the impact simple modifications may have for a person living with dementia. The app follows 10 Dementia Enabling Environment Principles which includes reducing visual stimulation to avoid causing stress, creating clear pathways free of obstacles and personalising areas with familiar objects.

Built for a tablet, the app is available on the App Store and Google Play Store [http://bit.ly/2dC2JNB].

twitter: @AlzheimersAus

Dementia Friendly Home

Alzheimer Scotland have developed a Dementia Friendly Home at BRE Innovation Park. The house highlights how adjustments to traditional properties could make living at home safer for the increasing number in the Scottish population who are being diagnosed with the condition annually.

website: www.alzscot.org/news_and_community/news/ 3621_dementia_friendly_home_unveiled_at_bre_innovation_park

Leisure and Pleasure

Arts 4 Dementia

Arts 4 Dementia are empowering people with memory loss through artistic stimulation. They work in partnership with organisations developing dance, music, art, drama and poetry activities helping to re-energise people in the early stages of dementia and their carers. Bridging a vital gap in care, their projects enable participants to restore creative skills and learn new ones, which rebuilds confidence, joy in social activity and a sense of achievement at each workshop.

website: www.arts4dementia.org.uk
facebook: www.facebook.com/Arts4Dementia
twitter: @Arts4Dementia

Dementia Dogs

Dementia Dogs are assistance dogs that help people with dementia lead more fulfilled, independent and stress-free lives.

A dog is paired with a person with dementia. The dog can help people with dementia maintain their waking, sleeping and eating routine, remind them to take medication, improve confidence, keep them active and engaged with their local community, as well as providing a constant companion who will reassure when facing new and unfamiliar situations.

website: www.dementiadog.org
facebook: www.facebook.com/dementiadogproject
twitter: @dementiadog

Dementia Adventure

Dementia Adventure connects people living with dementia with nature and a sense of adventure. Dementia Adventure offers short breaks and adventure holidays for people living with dementia. Whether people live in care homes or in their own home, Dementia Adventure offers everyone the opportunity to connect with nature and meet others in the local community. The enterprise also works alongside care providers, local authorities and health services to help them support people living with dementia to get out into nature as much as possible.

website: www.dementiaadventure.co.uk
facebook: www.facebook.com/DementiaAdventure
twitter: @DementiaAdv

Growing Support

Growing Support turns underused care home gardens into bustling hubs of community activity and thriving growing spaces. Studies show residents of care homes spend most of their time doing nothing and are twice as likely to feel lonely as people living in the community. Growing Support provides volunteer led, social and therapeutic gardening activities. This includes weekly gardening clubs, mostly in care home gardens, where people with dementia are enabled to grow their own food, exercise vital muscle groups, enjoy sensory stimulation, socialise and develop a renewed sense of purpose and achievement.

website: www.growingsupport.co.uk
facebook: www.facebook.com/GrowingSupport
twitter: @Growing_Support

Fidget Items

Fidget Items usually a quilt, twiddle or memory mitts have various items , including ribbons, buttons or beads patches attached to keep restless fingers busy, touching and playing with the items helping to reduce anxiety and promote calm. They help to stimulate curiosity, memories and awareness, provide a sense of purpose and of doing something, and have a calming effect for people living with Alzheimer's and dementia There are some wonderful examples of Fidget Items displayed on various Pinterest Boards.

pinterest: www.pinterest.com/pin/522206519276584569

Memory Mitts

An increasing number of hospital are encouraging keen knitters to make and send in special 'memory mitts' to support the care of patients with dementia in hospital. Poole Hospital have provided a pattern perfect for using up left over and odd balls of wool.

website: www.poole.nhs.uk/about-us/latest-news/2015-news/knit-a-mitt-for-patients.aspx

Engage & Create

Engage & Create is a not-for-profit organisation that uses creativity and conversation to improve the quality of life for people with dementia and those that care for them. The Ignite Programme offers a complete package of training, resources and support to help organisations provide cognitively stimulating activity for people with dementia. Created with the help of people with dementia, it improves wellbeing and helps people remain mentally active.

website: www.engageandcreate.com
facebook: www.facebook.com/engageandcreate
twitter: @engageandcreate

Remember Better

When I Paint narrated by Olivia de Havilland, is the first international documentary about the positive impact of art and other creative therapies for people with Alzheimer's and how these approaches can change the way we look at the disease. The DVD package includes the documentary as well as a series of short supplemental films that further highlight special programs and the how-tos of organizing an outing, a creative workshop or recreating social bonds between people with Alzheimer's and their families.

website: irememberbetterwhenipaint.wordpress.com
twitter: @IRememberBetter

Apps for Pleasure

There are many apps, tools and resources to support those living with dementia and their carers including apps designed for entertainment and relaxation. They can play a part in bringing back activities which participants have missed from their lives. Talk to people about activities they enjoy doing! Before downloading or buying an app it is worthwhile reading the Terms and Conditions of Use and checking reviews in the Apple or Google App Store.

Pigment

Pigment (free to download but with a Premium Access paid subscription) allows you to colour as you would on paper with actual coloured pencils. Choose from 350+ hand curated, professionally drawn illustrations, 8 different kinds of pencils, markers and brushes, and an unlimited number of colors to choose from. Completed artwork can be friends and family.

app store: itunes.apple.com/gb/app/pigment-coloring-book-for/
id1062006344?mt=8

Painterly

Painterly (£1.49) allows you to create beautiful evocative pictures even if you do not have advanced drawing skills or formal art · trainingAllows for painting with more than 60 virtual brushes, as well as importing photos and then painting them

app store: itunes.apple.com/gb/app/painterly/id451443771?mt=8

Imutt

Imutt (free but the Dogs Trust will invite a donation) This game from the Dogs Trust allows users to look after an impossibly cute virtual rescue dog for five days. Perfect and no need to walk in bad weather!

app store: itunes.apple.com/gb/app/imutt/id422054734?mt=8

FlowerGarden

FlowerGarden(free with further in-app purchases) allows you to pick virtual seeds, plant them, water them and watch them grow. This is especially significant for participants who used to enjoy growing plants and are missing their former gardens. A top-5 app on the iTunes App Store.

app store: itunes.apple.com/gb/app/flower-garden-free-grow-flowers/id327466677?mt=8

Memory and Brain Training

MindMate

MindMate is a free app to improve the self-management skills of those who live with dementia; support the person with dementia as well as the carer in his/her everyday life; and increase the quality of live for patients as well as carers.

MindMate helps you to train your brain and provides you with tools like reminders. If you need to, you can access advice about nutrition and exercises and learn more about dementia. The app supports you in living well with dementia, no matter if you are a caregiver, family member or someone diagnosed with dementia.

website: www.mindmate-app.com
facebook: www.facebook.com/mindmateapp
twitter: @MindMateApp

Memrica

Memrica Prompt is a service that helps anyone with memory problems make the most of each day. Designed to reduce the anxiety and frustration caused by forgetting essential information the app provides a visual diary, with images and background information included in reminders. Memrica can be built over time with photos, prompts, references and calendar notes to make all aspects of everyday life easier, such as going to the hairdresser or doctor, as well as relating to family and friends. It aims to maintain confidence and independence especially in the early stages of dementia. Memrica is currently being piloted and people are invited to sign up to test the Prompt app. There will be a subscription fee when the app is released commercially.

website: memricaprompt.com
facebook: www.facebook.com/memrica
twitter: @memrica

Reminiscence

Digital reminiscence therapy gives a new dynamic to traditional methods of reminiscence which provide prompts, such as photos, music or familiar items to encourage people to talk about their

memories and stimulate conversation. There is considerable
evidence to support the benefits of reminiscence for older people,
not just those living with dementia. Research shows that using
reminiscence therapy also creates a stronger bond between carers
and those cared for. Caregivers report a reduction in stress and
improved knowledge of their loved ones whilst helping them to
relive family moments and events.

Alive!

Alive! is a charity dedicated to improving the quality of life of older
people in care through meaningful activities. They enable older
people to shape the content and direction of Alive! sessions, which
include the use of new technology, guided reminiscence, creative,
energising and physical activities. Their vision is for a world where
all older people in care homes live with dignity and respect, access
to choices, their local communities, hobbies and interests, learning,
and meaningful activities. They believe identifying shared
experiences and interests creates a focus for conversation, helping
introverted, isolated people to join in and connect with both care
home staff and other residents.

website: aliveactivities.org
facebook: www.facebook.com/aliveactivities/timeline
twitter: @aliveactivities

Dementia Diaries

Dementia Diaries is a national project bringing together people's
experiences of living with dementia as a series of audio diaries.
It serves as a public record and a personal archive that documents
the day-to-day lives of people living with dementia, with the aim of
prompting a richer dialogue about the varied forms of the condition.

As the use of technology often becomes more difficult for those living with dementia, this project uses 3D printed mobile handsets which are customised to be as simple as possible allowing Dementia Diaries to both record audio diary entries and capture thoughts and experiences as they occur. These handsets are linked to a dedicated voicemail and as soon as a diary entry is recorded, it is automatically sent via the internet to the editorial team at On Our Radar. The team will then listen to it, transcribe it and curate it for publication.

website: www.dementiadiaries.org
facebook: www.facebook.com/dementiadiariesposts
twitter: @DementiaTweets

House of Memories

House of Memories is an award-winning training programme, run by the Museum of Liverpool, which targets the carers of people living with dementia. It provides participants with information about dementia and equips them with the practical skills and knowledge to facilitate a positive quality of life experience for people living with dementia. As part of the House of Memories programme the memory suitcase is a free loan service which contains objects, memorabilia and photographs to help engagement with the people being cared for. There is a free downloadable app which allows individuals to explore objects from the past and share memories and reminisce about a range of every day objects, from school life to sport. Objects can be saved to a personal memory tree, memory box or memory timeline. It can be used by anyone, but has been designed for, and with, people living with dementia and their carers. The app is available for iPhone, iPad and Android.

website: www.liverpoolmuseums.org.uk/learning/projects/house-of-memories/my-house-of-memories-app.aspx
twitter: @NML_Muse

Life Story Network

Life Story Network develop, deliver and promote improvements to the quality of care and support received by those who may be marginalised through ill-health, or social circumstance, by working closely with care providers, carers, housing associations, transport providers, schools and advocacy groups. Life Story Network are developing tide, 'together in dementia everyday' an involvement network that recognises family carers of people with dementia are experts by experience, experts that can play a significant role in supporting other carers, influencing policy and shaping improved responsive local commissioned services.

website: www.lifestorynetwork.org.uk
facebook: www.facebook.com/Life-Story-Network-CIC-162014757278346
twitter: @LifeStoryNetwrk

Memory Box Network

The Memory Box Network is a free to use social media based platform that enables people to easily upload and share memorable materials tailored for the person with dementia to help them remember past times which can stimulate their more recent memories and their cognitive abilities. Technology is being used to access to millions of online resources which include video clips, audio recordings of either spoken word or music, photographs, news clippings, letters and stories.

website: memoryboxnetwork.org
facebook: www.facebook.com/TheMemoryBoxNetwork
twitter: @TMBNet

My Own Memory Lane

My Own Memory Lane is a tool designed to assist the memory-impaired with remembering loved ones and significant memories. If you are the caregiver of someone who lives with a memory-impacting form of dementia such as Alzheimer's, they offer hosting of a custom website using images and captions that you provide. My Own Memory Lane will create a website for free and host it for one week so you can see if it will be beneficial. The subscription fee after the one week trial is $2.99 per month.

website: myownmemorylane.com
twitter: @MyOwnMemoryLane

Sporting Memories Network

Sporting Memories Network promotes and develops memories of sport with older fans to improve wellbeing through conversation and reminiscence. Sports reminiscence provides the opportunity to document a person's favourite sports events, teams and moments. Sporting memories provides an alternative focus for men who are reluctant to join in other group and reminiscence based activities. Sporting Memories are supported by an impressive range of star supporters from such diverse worlds as motor racing, football and cricket. Sporting Memories Network set an ambitious target on World Alzheimer's Day to share Bill's Story which eventually reached 12,500,000 people through the power of social media. Sporting Memories Network has been voted as the Best Football Community Scheme & the Best National Dementia Friendly Initiative

website: www.sportingmemoriesnetwork.com
facebook: www.facebook.com/SportingMemoriesNetwork
twitter: @SportsMemNet

Research and Engagement

involving people living with dementia and their carers

Alzheimer's Society

Alzheimer's Society is a pioneer in public involvement in dementia research. Their Research Network is a team of over 250 carers, former carers and people with dementia who are actively involved in shaping our Research programme.

website: www.alzheimers.org.uk/site/scripts/documents_info.php? documentID=110

Sea Hero Quest

Alzheimer's Research UK has teamed up with Deutsche Telekom and scientists from University College London and the University of East Anglia to develop Sea Hero Quest, a smartphone game that re-writes the rules on how we go about dementia research. Sea Hero Quest is a mobile game which contributes to research on dementia. One of the first symptoms of dementia is loss of navigational skills. Doctors cannot differentiate between getting lost caused by disease and getting lost caused by natural ageing because a benchmark of "normal" does not exist. The game puts you in the shoes of an unnamed sailor, whose father is slowly losing memories of his life as a seafaring explorer. To try and help him remember his past, your job is to travel around cartoon waterways in search of pieces of his old journal. At the start of a level, you're given a top-down map of the waterways that shows a number of buoy markers you need to navigate through. Once you've memorised it, you simply need to sail your ship around the 3D world and hit each buoy in numerical order. The information about the route you take, and what you do if you get lost, is saved and transmitted for further analysis. This will inform new approaches towards dementia diagnosis and management.

website: www.alzheimersresearchuk.org/our-research/what-we-do/
sea-hero-quest
facebook: www.facebook.com/AlzheimersResearchUK
twitter: @ARUKnews

Dementia Citizens

Dementia Citizens is a new digital platform that connects people affected by dementia and researchers. Using apps on smartphones and tablets, people with dementia and carers can enjoy activities that also contribute to dementia research. Current apps available are Book of You a life story book to share happy memories with carers, friends and family and Playlist for Life to enjoy personal music with carers, friends and family.

Dementia Citizens offers a range of tools for researchers which will make it easier to carry out dementia research. Join Dementia Research and Dementia Citizens are partners in promoting active engagement in dementia research

website: dementiacitizens.org
research website: dementiacitizens.org/researchers

Join dementia research

Join dementia research is a place to register your interest in participating in dementia research. Anyone, with or without dementia, can register as a volunteer or sign-up for someone else, providing that they have their consent.

website: www.joindementiaresearch.nihr.ac.uk
twitter: @beatdementia

BRACE

BRACE raise funds to support dementia research and award grants to university-based researchers in South West England and South Wales. The Our policy of funding research only within a region of the UK is pragmatic, not parochial and a sensible policy for a charity which does not have the financial or staff resources of the big funders.

Useful information is provided about their achievements and impact including the development of an assessment tool, Bristol Activities of Daily Living Scale (BADLS) which is used worldwide to assist in the diagnosis of dementia

website: www.alzheimers-brace.org
facebook: www.facebook.com/BRACEAlzheimersResearch
twitter: @AlzheimersBRACE

Talking Mats

Talking Mats is a visual communication framework that allows people with communication difficulties to think about an issue and express their views. They have developed a number of useful resources which are free to anyone working with people with communication disability.

Talking Mats are collaborating with @PatientOpinion to help people with dementia share their stories

website: www.talkingmats.com
twitter: @TalkingMats

Patient Opinion

Patient Opinion was founded in 2005 and is now the UK's leading independent non-profit feedback platform for health services. Patient Opinion encourages honest and meaningful conversations between patients and health services and they believe that individual stories can help make health services better.

website: www.patientopinion.org.uk
facebook: www.facebook.com/patientopinion
twitter: @patientopinion

Robots and the Internet of Things

There is considerable interest and investment in the potential of robots and the Internet of Things (IoT) to support people living with dementia and their carers. The use of companion robots and assistive technology in care for older people is not widespread but now the government have launched the UK's first official robotics strategy this is likely to lead to an increased use of robots in our everyday lives. There are increasing calls for more public debate on the ethical dimensions of using robots in health and care.

Paro

Paro is an interactive robot which allows the benefits of animal therapy to be made available to people in hospitals and care homes where live animals would present treatment or logistical difficulties. PARO has been in use in Japan and throughout Europe since 2003. PARO has five kinds of sensors: tactile, light, audition, temperature, and posture sensors, with which it can perceive people and its environment. With the light sensor, PARO can recognize light and dark. He feels being stroked and beaten by tactile sensor, or being held by the posture sensor. PARO can learn to behave in a way that the user prefers, and to respond to its new name. By interaction with people, PARO responds as if it is alive, moving its head and legs and making sounds by imitating the voice of a real baby harp seal. There are about 3,000 Paro seals worldwide, the vast majority in Japan and around 10 in the UK; The effectiveness of the robotic seal in a dementia care setting is now being evaluated in a joint project involving Sheffield Health and Social Care NHS Foundation Trust and the University of Sheffield.

website: www.parorobots.com

Mark Brown has shared his thoughts and experiences when he met Paro the seal in his post "On falling in love with a robot"

blog: medium.com/@MarkOneinFour/on-falling-in-love-with-a-robot-a047e8cb6b73#.mfmtɪnvqa
twitter: @MarkOneinFour

Potentially the Internet of Things (IoT) could support older or disabled people to manage their home with the minimum of help by sending warnings or requests for support to family members or other carers. A big challenge is to encourage designers, manufacturers and app developers to ensure that digital products are inclusive and accessible to everyone who may benefit from them.

Some examples:

Amazon Echo

Amazon Echo is a hands-free speaker you control with your voice. Echo connects to the Alexa Voice Service(AVS) to play music, provide information, news, sports scores, weather, and more instantly. 'All you have to do is ask'. Designed for your home, it is plugged into the mains and connected to your wifi.It's been on sale to the general public in the USA since last summer and is now available in the UK.

In his post 'Managing our health: One conversation' at a time Maneesh Juneja provides case studies showing how Amazon Echo can support people living with dementia.

website: maneeshjuneja.com/blog/2016/9/17/health-conversations
twitter: @ManeeshJuneja

Alcove

Alcove is pioneering independent living and revolutionising care and support through an IoT digital care service which enables older and disabled adults to remain living independently in their own homes. The award-winning service brings together technologies that work, look great and are easy to use to help care providers save money, enhance safeguarding and improve quality of life. Alcove enables remote monitoring to check on loved ones giving them continued independence while providing reassurance to the family.

website: www.youralcove.com
facebook: www.facebook.com/youralcove
twitter: @youralcove

Specialist Design, Advice and Shops

Whilst the consumer market for technology is relatively underdeveloped some dementia charities now have online shops and there are examples of specialist organisations selling products online to help people with dementia and their families make more informed decisions about the use of technology.

Disabled Living Foundation

The Disabled Living Foundation (DLF) is a national charity providing impartial advice, information and training on independent living. DLF offers an unparalleled range of information on daily living equipment and other useful advice for people who might need some help in living their live to the full. The Helpline 0300 999 0004 available weekdays 10-4pm offers free, impartial advice about mobility products or other types of daily living equipment for older and disabled people.

website: www.dlf.org.uk

AskSARA

AskSARA is an award-winning online guided advice tool about support for daily living

website: asksara.dlf.org.uk
facebook: www.facebook.com/dlfuk
twitter: @DLFUK

Active Minds

Active Minds is an award-winning product design company who create and sell meaningful activity products for people with dementia. Active Minds hopes that by providing meaningful and engaging activities for nursing and residential homes it will help reduce problems of depression, boredom and isolation so commonly associated with dementia.

website: active-minds.co.uk/our-products
twitter: @ActiveMindsUK

AT Dementia

AT Dementia are a charity who provide information and advice on assistive technologies that can help people with dementia live more independently. The AT Guide is an online self-assessment support tool to help people with dementia and their carers make informed decisions about the use of assistive technology to support independence. Customers are encouraged to share their experiences with others through reviews.

website: www.atdementia.org.uk
facebook: www.facebook.com/atdementia
twitter: @ATDementia

Designability

Designability is a national charity who research and develop assistive technologies to transform lives. They are engineering and design experts with a passion for creating life-changing assistive technologies who conduct original research and develop products that meet real needs. They advocate better technology for everyone and believe inclusive design is the only way forward.

Dementia products include the: Day Clock, Ward Orientation Clock, Simple Music Player, One Button Digital Radio, One Button Analogue Radio and Wander Reminder

website: www.designability.org.uk
facebook: www.facebook.com/DesignabilityUK
twitter: @DesignabilityUK

Unforgettable

Unforgettable aims to improve the lives of those living with memory loss and dementia by bringing together specially selected products together with practical advice and a supportive and sharing community. The company was founded through personal experience and passion to help people live well with dementia. The Unforgettable marketplace offers an increasingly diverse range of products and services specifically selected to address the daily challenges of those affected by dementia.

website: www.unforgettable.org
facebook: www.facebook.com/unforgettable.org
twitter: @Unforget_org

Technology Enabled Care (TECs)

Technology enabled careservices* (TECS) such as telecare and telehealth, can be life-changing not only for the individual, but for family, carers and the professionals involved in their care.Dementia makes aspects of day-to-day life more difficult for the person living with the condition. There is increasing recognition that devices and technologies can make life easier for people with dementia and their carers. To list all the telecare and telehealth resources would require a separate book. The following organisations provide useful information and advice about assistive technologies and developments.

Alzheimer's Society

Alzheimer's Society have published a useful guide to Assistive Technology and devices to help with everyday living which can be downloaded from the website.

website: www.alzheimers.org.uk/site/scripts/documents_info.php?documentID=109

AbilityNet

AbilityNet offers expert information and services on technology and disability. They specialise in assistive technology for computers, as well as offering help in using mainstream computers in the most accessible way possible. The My Computer My Way is the AbilityNet's interactive service to help adapt a computer to individual needs. AbilityNet provides a range of support to help disabled and older people get the most from their home computers, tablets and smartphones. AbilityNet can provide advice about technology and disability on 0800 269 545 Monday – Friday, during office hours.

website: www.abilitynet.org.uk
facebook: www.facebook.com/AbilityNet
twitter: @AbilityNet

AT Home campaign

The AT Home campaign is a collaboration amongst the 14 Local Authorities covering the West Midlands, supported by companies who operate in this market. The campaign aims to encourage people to think about how independent living and mobility equipment, also known as assistive technology, can help you, or someone you care for, to continue to live independently in a healthy and safe environment at home.

Research has consistently confirmed that awareness of assistive technology is very low, held back by a combination of factors. A recent study led by Coventry University found that 60% of consumers questioned said that lack of awareness was a barrier to greater use/purchase of assistive technology. However the same research also found that 85% felt that the costs of purchasing were worth it given that it would make life easier*. This demonstrates that people are willing to consider paying, from their own pockets, for products and services, provided that they feel it will help.

website: www.athome.uk.com

NHS Choices

NHS Choices provides guidance on Telecare and alarms

website: www.nhs.uk/conditions/social-care-and-support-guide/pages/telecare-alarms.aspx

Rica

Rica is the trading name of the national research charity Research Institute for Consumer Affairs who focus specifically on issues of concern to disabled and older consumers. Rica was founded through Consumers Association, publishers of Which? but is now an independent charity. With grant funding they research and publish free consumer reports. They are all based on rigorous research and provide practical information needed by disabled and older consumers. They offer useful consumer guides to technology to help make home life easier, household appliances that are easy to use and products for personal care, including a guide to bathing products and medicine boxes and dispensers.

website: www.rica.org.uk
facebook: www.facebook.com/RicaUK
twitter: @RicaUK

New Dynamics of Ageing Programme

The New Dynamics of Ageing Programme is an eight year multidisciplinary research initiative with the ultimate aim of improving the quality of life of older people. The programme was a unique collaboration between five UK Research Councils and the largest and most ambitious research programme on ageing ever mounted in the UK. Of particular interest is the mappmal project developing prototypes for the prevention of malnutrition in older people and the NDA Handbook. The Handbook is intended as a guide to the research outcomes for a lay audience, and particularly for older people and their organisations. It aims to put the new evidence and new insights generated through the research into the hands of older people themselves, so that they can make use of this information to spread new knowledge, to campaign, and to influence policy and practice.

website: www.newdynamics.group.shef.ac.uk
twitter: @NDAProgramme

Telecare Learning and Improvement Network

The Telecare Learning and Improvement Network (Telecare Lin) is the national network supporting local service redesign for people through the application of telecare and telehealth to aid the delivery of housing, health, social care and support services for older and vulnerable people. Telecare LIN provides a free monthly eNewsletter with extensive curated coverage of digital health and technology enabled care references from the UK and around the world including telehealth, telecare, mobile health, telemedicine, ehealth, smart home technologies and Internet of Things. An invaluable resource for keeping up to date with the latest developments in health informatics (including electronic health and care records), big data, artificial intelligence and health and care robotics.

website: www.telecarelin.org.uk
twitter: @clarkmike

TSA

TSA (formerly known as Telecare Services Association) is the industry body for Technology Enabled Care (TEC), representing the largest industry specific network in Europe. TSA works across health, housing and social care through a wide range of public services (NHS, local authorities, Fire and Rescue Services), housing associations, leading industry suppliers, independent and voluntary sector organisations. TSA promotes and supports the technology enabled care industry, highlighting the benefits of TEC for commissioners across health and social care, service users, their family and carers.

TSA Find a Service can help with telecare, telehealth or other technology enabled service needs. TSA Integrated Code of Practice encourages organisations to become quality accredited for technology enabled services, including telecare and/or telehealth.

website: www.tsa-voice.org.uk
twitter: @TSAVoice

Examples of technology enabled care include:

Just Checking

Just Checking is an easy-to-use online activity monitoring system that helps people stay independent in their own home.

The system is easy to install, simple to use with discreet wireless motion sensors and a plug-in controller this creates a clear summary of daily living activity that can be viewed securely online. Just Checking will give an insight into how best to provide support for a family member who lives alone, particularly if they are becoming forgetful.

website: www.justchecking.co.uk
facebook: www.facebook.com/justchecking

Canary

Canary is a discreet, easy to install monitoring and notification system that provides round the clock reassurance to family members whilst allowing the older person to stay in the home they love.Canary respects the privacy of people who need care and support so does not use cameras so no-one can be seen or heard.

website: www.canarycare.co.uk
facebook: www.facebook.com/Canary-537691109672841
twitter: @canary_care

Buddi

Buddi is a personal locating device that uses GPS technology to accurately calculate its location (like an in-car Sat Nav), and the mobile phone network to communicate that location to secure computers. Every user is provided with unique details to log onto the Buddi website to access their Buddi account and to carry out location requests.

website: www.buddi.co.uk
facebook: www.facebook.com/buddiltd
twitter: @buddi_gps

Vega GPS Watch

The Vega GPS Watch is a purpose built system to aid safer walking for those with Alzheimer or other cognitive disorders. Vega allows wearers to walk freely in a predetermined safe zone but raises an automatic alarm should the wearer walk outside of this zone. Vega also features an RF home base that indicates to the Vega bracelet that the wearer is at home.

website: www.tunstallemergencyresponse.ie/vega
facebook: www.facebook.com/TunstallER
twitter: @tunstaller

Conclusions

Surprisingly there is no shortage of innovations in digital technology and millions of pounds are being spent supporting further developments. But there is a huge information gap and no strategic approach to embedding digital technology in the range of options to support people with dementia to live more fulfilling lives.

Information, advice and advocacy are essential in enabling people to make choices about their care and support needs. Care recipients, their families and carers need signposts to explore what technology products and services are available, both through statutory services or to purchase independently. There are an increasing number of web and mobile based applications from simple information to more complex care management tools that will transform the delivery of social care.

The aim of the Click Guide is to ensure that people living with dementia, their carers, families, friends and professionals involved in adult social care can keep up to date with developments in the digital world, I hope you will be encouraged to share your thoughts and contribute to the many conversations about improving dementia services which now happen every day.

Finally, my thanks to family, friends and colleagues who have generously supported the development of the Click Guide to Dementia Resources.

Index

www.ingramcontent.com/pod-product-compliance
Lightning Source LLC
Chambersburg PA
CBHW070304290526
45791CB00003B/1076